The Insomniac's ABZzzzzzz Book

With Quotations from William Shakespeare

Jeffrey Haseltine, Ph.D.

ISBN-10: 1517225728
ISBN-13: 978-1517225728

Dedication

For all those who just can't get to sleep.

Introduction

This book is supposed to put you to sleep.

I've scoured dictionaries for the most boring words in the English language. Words that don't have any connotation whatsoever: nothing positive, nothing negative, zero effect on your blood pressure. These are words that were carefully chosen to take you nowhere, relate to nothing, stir no emotions: no politics, no religion, no controversy, no excitement, no beauty or ugliness, joy or sorrow, good or bad. Just soporific blandness. An alphabetical college lecture.

The challenge you face as an insomniac is that your brain just won't shut down at night. You keep fretting about ghosts from the past, or the present, or even the future. And every image, emotion, sound, or word that you conjure up to dispel those ghosts just makes things worse. Everything seems to be connected to something else, which leads you back to stress, a heightened pulse, and despair borne of another night with only a few hours of sleep. My desire is to cure your insomnia, or at least get you through one night, by filling your mind with dullness. So settle back and have a good read. No, wait—not a good read, just a passive, boring, mind-numbing, nodding-off read.

Here's a book that you just can't wait to put down.

About the Shakespeare Quotes

As Horatio held the dying Hamlet in his arms, he gave us a line you'll recall from long ago: "Good night, sweet prince: And flights of angels sing thee to thy rest!"

That's a pretty dramatic send-off, and involves a deeper kind of "rest" than we're seeking here, but it reminds me that William Shakespeare is a good source of comforting sleepy-time admonitions. So if the ABZZZZ lists themselves aren't enough to set you snoring, maybe hearing from a variety of Elizabethan well-wishers will help.

I didn't include the usual citations for the quotations—just the names of the speakers—because I didn't want to clutter your brain with anything intriguing. You'll recognize some of these folks, and not others, but that doesn't matter. Just "rest" assured (yes, that's a pun) that even characters from Shakespeare's centuries-old tales are interested in helping you get a good night's sleep.

So don't try to drag up the contexts for these comforting quotations. Just take them at face value and let Shakespeare's words do for you now what they likely did for you back in high school—bear you off on wings of angels to a pleasant sleep.

" Would I were sleep and peace, so sweet to rest!"

-Romeo

A

aardvark abaft abalone
abattoir abbot abloom
aboard abode about abridge
academic accede acceptor
accordion accretion acorn
adapters additively adequate
adobe aegis aerator
aesthete affably affinity
afield agglomeration agleam
agora ahem alpaca alveoli
amalgam amble ambrosia
amoeba angularity annals
annotate appendage arbitrary
arcane ashbin asterisk

"*Thou art inclined to sleep; 'tis a good dulness . . .*"

   —Prospero

B

backrest bade baffler bag
bagatelle baggages balsam
bakehouse balsam bangles
baobab bargepole barley
basketry bauble bead bean
bearers beeches beeswax
beige belays bendings berber
betoken biennial bilge
birched blah bland blank
blat bluish bluffer bodkin
boffin borax bored boron
bovine bream brine broccoli
bromide broth brown
bullion burble buttercup

" I would it were my fault to sleep
so soundly."

   -Brutus

C

cabbage cadge caftan
calico caliper canapé
canter capstan carafe
carbuncle cardigan carry
category cauliflower celery
chicory circa cirrus
clavicle climes clod cloud
cogs composite concept
confluence conifer context
continual cooker cooper
cordial corduroy coterie
couscous cowslips
crannies crinkly crocus
curator curlew cyclical

" O weary night, o long and tedious night . . . "

   -Helena

D

dabble daffodil daisy
dampers dateline daubed
deadpan decagon decimal
declension deemed deepish
defunct deluxe denim depot
devoid digestible dimmer
disband dishes dither ditty
divan docking doffed doily
dolomite doodle doorknob
dot dowel doze drab
drawer drawn drift droll
droned droplet drowsy
dubbed dulcimer dull
duration dustpan dwellers

" Now, good my lord, lie here and rest awhile."

–Kent

E

each ear earls earthworks
easel easterly eave eclectic
eddies effects effortless
egret eiderdown eightfold
elaborates elapses elbow
elderberries eleven elide
elongated elude emblem
eminent emitter emulsifies
encase endive endorsed
enigmas ensconced ensuing
entailed entropy enumerated
envoys eons epoch ergot
esters euphonium eventual
ewe expanse extend eyelet

" I'll pray, and then I'll sleep."

-King Lear

F

fabric faceplate facsimile
factual fairly familiar
fancifully far fascia fated
fauna feasibility feathers
featured fedora fellows
fennel ferromagnetic festal
fictional fife figs filler
finch finisher firsthand
fjords flange flaxen fledge
fluctuating flux flyweight
focusing fold folklorists
footpath forays forestry
formless forsythia fourth
frangipani fuchsia furze

" You are for dreams and slumbers,
brother . . ."

    -Troilus

G

gabardine gainers galleon
gammon garb garment gate
gazetteer gelled generalize
genotype geodesic gerbils
germane get gibbet gibbous
girders glazier glebe globes
glyphs gnu goblet gofer
golliwog good-natured gorse
governorship gracing gradient
gramophone grandly granite
graphologists gravel graze
greenery gripper grommets
groundwork grower grunter
guardedly guesses guideline

" *Thou quiet soul, sleep thou a quiet sleep . . .* "

  -Ghost of Lady Anne

H

haberdasher haddock hadron
halibut halves hams handy
hankering happen harbinger
hardiness hardwood harks
harrier hasp hatch hatters
haziness headrest hearable
heartening heather hedgehog
helmsman helpful heptagon
herewith hermetically heron
hexagonal hickory hinges
hob hocks hoist homage
homing homogeneous honed
honorific hoop horizontal
huddling hulled humdrum

" I have not slept one wink."

-Pisanio

I

ibex icebox icons ideas
ideograms idyllic igneous
ilk illogic illusion image
imaginable imbalances imbue
imitative immediateness
imminent impartial impasse
impassive impel imperfectly
impersonal impervious
imprint impulse inadvisability
inasmuch inaudible inboard
inch inclined incur indent
indeterminate indubitably
ingathered iridium ironing
irrespectively italics itself

" *God give your grace good rest!* "

-Brakenbury

J

jabbering jackdaws jackets
jadedly jailing jamboree
jambs jangling jargon
jaundiced jauntier jawline
jays jejunum jellied jennets
jerboas jerkins jestingly
jetsam jetties jiffy jingled
jocularity john joiners
jointed jollify jostling
joules journaling jowls
judders judicature juncture
juniper junker jurisdictional
jurist jussive justifiability
jute jutted juxtapose

" O sleep, O gentle sleep,

Nature's soft nurse . . ."

—King Henry IV

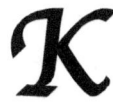

K

kaftan kale karma katydid
kebab keel keener keeper
kelp keratin kerchief kernel
kerning kettleful keying
kibitz kick-started killjoy
kilns kilobyte kilohertz
kilojoules kinase kindlier
kinematics kinetically kingly
kinked kinsman kippers
kitchenware kith kitsch
kiwis klaxon kloof knack
knee-deep knew knitting
knoll kookaburra krall krill
kudu kudzu kwachas

" Get thee to bed, and rest; for thou hast need."

-Lady Capulet

L

label laborious lacework
lachrymal lackadaisical
lackluster laconically lade
ladled ladybird laggards laird
laminated lamppost landfall
landholdings lapel lapsed
laryngitis latecomer laths
lattices leached learnable
leavings leftovers legato
leguminous lemmings lens
levels levers levied lexeme
lidless lifter ligature liken
listlessly loafers locations
lubber lumpen lumpish lur

"The sweetest sleep, and fairest-
boding dreams

That ever enter'd in a drowsy head."

    -Richmond

M

macaw macrophage madras
magnanimity magnetodynamics
mailable mainbrace maize
mallard managerially mandible
manganese marginalization
marmoset martinet mash
mawkish maypole meanders
medulla meeter memento
mention merely meridian
midafternoon midge mildew
mild-mannered mind miosis
miscellaneous modal mohair
molybdenum moorhen moot
mulberry munch murmured

" You were best to go to bed and
dream again . . ."

—Warwick

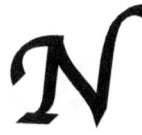

N

nameable narration narwhal
nasturtium nattering nearby
neaten nebular neckband
nectar needlecraft neighbor
neither neologism neoprene
nestable nethermost nettles
newfangled newt nibblers
niche niftily nimbleness
nimbus ninefold nocturnally
nod nodal nodular noggin
noiselessly nomenclatures
nominal nonentity noodles
noonday normalcy normed
nuclei nudged null numb

"*Dream on, dream on . . .*"

-Ghost of Buckingham

O

oatcakes obediently objects
obligingly oblong observatory
obsidian obtained occasional
occupational occur oceanic
ochre octagonal oculists
oddity offered offshoot
oh ohm okapi once one
onyx opacity operationally
opossum opted optionally
orange orderliness organza
orienteering ornamental
orthorhombic oscillated
osmium otherwise outer
outgrowths oval overlaid

" My soul is heavy, and I fain would sleep."

-Clarence

P

pachyderm packable paddock
paginate pails paintbox
pairing palaver palette
palindromic paling paneling
paperweight papyri parabolic
paraffin parallel parsed
parsnips pavement peachier
pebble peccary pedals peg
pendulum penny phenotype
philatelist phlebotomy phyla
pickings pin pinafore pinion
planks plop plover plurals
polka polyglot poplar posit
product prunes puffballs

" Sleep sound . . ."

-Puck

Q

quack quacked quackers
quacking quackish quacks
quadrangle quadrilaterals
quadrille quadruped quaff
quaggas quagmire quaintly
quaintness qualitatively
qualms quantifiably quark
quarries quart quarterstaff
quarto quartzite quash
quatrain quayside quelled
queried querulously queue
quiche quid quill quince
quinine quintets quoits
quorum quotable quoter

" And then with what haste you can get you to bed."

-Simonides

R

radishes raffia ragamuffins
ragbag ragout ragwort
raiment raisin rambled ramp
randomization rarebit rasher
raspy rather readable ready
reappear reared reassembled
rebus recap recede recent
recluse recoup rectory
redo reed referent regimen
regular rehash remuneration
repaint repast resin retails
rheumatism rhododendron
rhubarb ripples rookery
roundish rubidium ruminate

" Get you to bed again; it is not day."

    –Brutus

S

sachet saddlebags salient
salubrious salver sameness
sapling sartorial satchels
satisfactorily saucepans
sauerkraut saunter scalable
scentless schwa scoreless
sedans seldom semicolons
sensible sepia sequel shale
shapeless shelving shinbone
shoebox shopkeeper shrank
siding sieve silt sixpence
slack slosh sludge slushy
smithy snippet snooze so
solenoid sparse stumped

" I hate a man who goes to sleep at once; there is a sort of indefinable something about it which is not exactly an insult, and yet is an insolence."

—Mark Twain (just seeing if you're still awake)

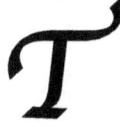

tablespoon tactical talc
tame teabag technicalities
teleconference telegraphy
telex tenable tend tendrils
tepid tertiary textile than
thatched thaw thenceforth
thesauri thimbleful thirds
throaty thyme tibia timidity
tinker toaster tokens tonal
tootle topical topologists
tortoise torus totem tout
trademark trail transactions
transient transpire trawling
trestle trot truncate tubs

" And sleep, that sometimes shuts
up sorrow's eye,

Steal me awhile from mine own
company."

-Helena

u

unacquainted unadventurous
unambitious unarticulated
unassertive unassuming
unattributable uncertainties
uncommitted unconfirmed
undefined undetermined
undistinguished unemotional
unenthusiastically unexcited
uninspiring unmotivated
unobservant unoriginal
unquantifiable unrefrigerated
unremarkable unscheduled
unscientific unsensational
unspectacular unsubstantial

" Sing me now asleep . . ."

-Titania

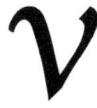

V

vacated vacillating vacuous
vague valance validate valise
valves vane vantage vapid
vaporous variants variously
vary vat vectored veering
veldt vellum velodrome vend
veneer ventilation verbalized
verisimilitude vermillion
versification vertically vests
vicariously viceroy vicinities
viewfinder vignette villagers
vintner vinyl viola virtually
vocalization vole vouchsafe
vulcanize vulpine vying

" Get thee to bed."

-Macbeth

W

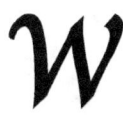

waders waft wagged wagon
wainscot waiver walkways
wallchart walnuts wapiti
warrens washbasin waters
waxworks wearisome weave
wedge well-wishers wending
westbound wheelbarrow
whereabouts wherewithal
wicket wide-ranging widths
windfall windsock winging
wombats wont woodlouse
woolen workable worsted
would wrappings wrens
writings wrongdoings wryly

" Good night, good night! as sweet repose and rest

Come to thy heart as that within my breast!"

-Juliet

X

ex-actuarial science teacher

ex-call center representative

ex-campaign manager

ex-commodities trader

ex-customer care rep

ex-deputy general manager

ex-fabric sales clerk

ex-loan application specialist

ex-network technician

ex-payroll administrator

ex-regulations monitor

ex-savings and loan teller

ex-tax accountant

ex-xylophonist

"To sleep; perchance to dream . . ."

-Hamlet

Y

yak yawn yam yawn yaps
yawn yard yawn yardage
yawn yardsticks yawner
yarn yawn yarns yawn yaw
yawn ye yawn yeah yawn
yearlong yawn yea yawn
yellowed yawn yellowish
yawn yeoman yawn yawns
yesterdays yawn yield yawn
yodeled yawn yogi yawn
yoked yawn yolks yawning
yonder yawn yore yawned
subliminal suggestion yawns
yawn yawner yawniest

"To bed, to bed: sleep kill those
pretty eyes,

And give as soft attachment to thy
senses

As infants' empty of all thought!"

   -Troilus

"And so, good rest."

   -Silvia

Z

zappy

zzealot

zzzebus

zzzzeniths

zzzzzeolite

zzzzzzephyr

zzzzzzzeppelin

zzzzzzzzeroed

zzzzzzzzzetas

zzzzzzzzzzigzag

zzzzzzzzzzzincs

zzzzzzzzzzzzither

zzzzzzzzzzzzzoning

zzzzzzzzzzzzzzzooplankton

Other Shakespeare quotation books by Jeffrey Haseltine:

**How to Cheat at Cribbage—With Quotations from
   William Shakespeare**

**Shakespeare Quotation Cryptograms—
   100 challenging puzzles to test your decoding
   skills and brush up your Shakespeare**

The Complete Shakespeare's Ass Coloring Book